Table of Contents

INTRODUCTION

Women over 50 can face struggles when trying to lose weight. This can stem from several things. The main culprit is often a slowed metabolism. The leaner muscle you have, the faster your metabolism is. But as we get older, we lose lean muscle mass, and we often become less active than before. The result? Stubborn body fat that just won't seem to budge.

Intermittent fasting has become popular in recent years due to its range of health benefits and the fact that it does not restrict your food choices. Research shows that fasting can improve your metabolism, mental health, and possibly prevent some cancers. It can also ward off certain muscle, nerve, and joint disorders which can affect women over 50.

Intermittent fasting can provide significant health benefits if it is done right. Plus, an intermittent fasting meal plan can save you time and money. Personalized meal plans for intermittent fasting will allow you to:

- ★ Enjoy delicious food

- ★ Lose weight with less hunger
- ★ See fast results

There are over 25 delicious and nutritious recipes with everything you need to know about them, mention it; is it the ingredients? the directions of preparation? Or the nutritional information? All are contained in this book. I know you would not want only women over 50 to enjoy these recipes alone. The go-to meals are for everyone; old and young, women and men. You too need to lose weight and live a healthy lifestyle!

CHAPTER ONE
FROM START TO MIDDLE

What Is Intermittent Fasting

Intermittent fasting is a time-restricted diet where you switch from fasting to eating. There are many ways to do it, but ultimately, you are focusing on time windows rather than the foods you eat.

The concept builds on our prehistoric ancestors, who went long periods between hunting and eating. They also got much more activity than we do presently. In theory, following a similar eating pattern as early humans can reduce the risk of high blood pressure, obesity, and heart disease.

Some proponents claim that intermittent fasting helps the body achieve ketosis. During this state, the body lacks carbs and instead will burn fat and turn it into fuel, encouraging fat loss and giving you more energy. Sounds pretty good, right?

Intermittent fasting (IF) involves cycling between periods of fasting and eating — and it has recently become very popular. Intermittent fasting is not something unusual but a part of everyday, normal life. It is perhaps the oldest and most powerful dietary intervention imaginable.

What Does Research Say About Intermittent Fasting for Women Over 50

In an article by the Journal of Mid-Life Health, different researches were accumulated in order to delineate the role of intermittent fasting in women's health, especially those in their mid-age. In simpler words, intermittent fasting refers to adjusting your eating schedule in such a way that you divide the periods of eating and fasting during the course of a day. The research shows that fasting for women over 50 has several health benefits that include weight loss, improved physical health, and sound mental health. To explain further, let us delve into the physical, medical, and mental health aspects of intermittent fasting separately.

Physical and Medical Benefits of Intermittent Fasting

Studies regarding the therapeutic role of intermittent fasting have come up with multiple health benefits that are associated with fasting for women over 50. Following are the significant changes that intermittent fasting can bring to your physical health, according to medical evidence:

Weight Loss: Weight loss is not the only benefit of intermittent fasting. Fasting is a practice that dates back to ancient times, and in some cultures is still practiced regularly.

Health benefits are a pleasant side effect of intermittent fasting, and many of those perks can affect women's health specifically.

Helps with Obesity and Belly Fat

The first and foremost health benefit that has attracted a vast majority of women into intermittent fasting is its effectiveness in helping to lose belly fat, the most stubborn and unhealthy fat that is accumulated around the abdomen.

Musculoskeletal Health. This includes conditions like osteoporosis, arthritis, and lower back pain. Fasting has been shown to promote hormone secretion from the thyroid. This can promote bone health and help prevent bone fractures.

Metabolic Health: Some women go through menopause in their 50s. Menopause can cause changes in your body that increase belly fat, insulin, and glucose. Fasting can help you decrease your blood pressure, cholesterol, and belly fat, which can improve insulin sensitivity. Fasting can also keep your metabolism on track as you age.

Supports Bone Minerals

An interesting discovery made by researchers regarding the favorable aspects of intermittent fasting indicates that fasting affects the way your body produces hormones. The hormones stir healthy changes to bone minerals such as calcium and phosphate, which reveals that it can lead to improved bone health.

Helps to Prevent Serious Diseases

Fasting has also proven to have a beneficial impact on the body's ability to fight diseases as serious as cancer. The practice of fasting activates certain processes in the body that indicate a decrease in the growth of tumor and cancer cells. This domain of health benefits of intermittent fasting is still under rigorous research to prove how optimally this method works for combating cancer.

Supports Good Reproductive Health

Intermittent fasting is also a safe and efficient way to improve your reproductive health in women. It has proved to be effective in treating the symptoms of PCOS (Polycystic Ovarian Syndrome), a condition that results in weight gain, irregular menstrual cycle, excess production of male testosterone, and imbalanced hormones. The condition mainly leads to infertility in women, and if aggravated, PCOS can also cause heart diseases and even cancer. Therefore, the significance or intermittent fasting can be proven through its role in treating reproductive illnesses.

Mental Health Aspects of Intermittent Fasting

Intermittent fasting not only benefits the body but is also a great mental health enhancer. Women in their fifties experience menopausal transition, the majority of who experience unpleasant symptoms throughout the process.

The mental impacts on women during this phase include irritability, moodiness, anxiety, tension, night sweat, and emotional instability. To curb these symptoms and allow healthy menopause, studies suggest that fasting is one natural, effective way to promote mental wellness during menopause. Intermittent fasting for women over 50 can help positively impact their mental health in the following ways:

- ★ It improves their mood and self-esteem
- ★ Decreases anxiety and stress
- ★ Fasting helps to reduce the symptoms of depression and improves social functioning
- ★ It is shown to have a positive impact on mood and increases vigilance

As a result of the positive mental effects of fasting, a sense of peacefulness, alacrity in mood, and boost in self-esteem can be achieved even if you are in your fifties. What else do we want, right? A peaceful existence is the biggest of blessings.

Other proven benefits of IF include:

- Tissue health
- Physical performance
- Heart health

Who Should Not Try Intermittent Fasting

Intermittent fasting is not for everyone. You should always check with your doctor before trying a new diet, even one that is proven to be beneficial. The following groups of people should avoid intermittent fasting:

- Children under the age of 18
- People with a history of eating disorders
- Pregnant and breastfeeding women

Keto Vs. Intermittent Fasting

Isn't that the ketogenic diet? Not exactly; the diets are different, but they have parallel benefits. Keto prohibits specific foods, while Intermittent Fasting focuses on healthy eating during certain times.

Evidence supports that the diet can help in losing weight, so how does it work?

Ultimately, the concept is not strict when it comes to eating a well-rounded diet of whole foods. The goal is to restructure precisely when you eat food rather than what you eat.

Mainly, you do not eat or drink anything (besides water and zero-calorie drinks) while fasting. Then, when it is time to eat, you will load up on low-carb, healthy foods like:

- Complex carbohydrates
- Lean proteins
- Fruits and veggies
- Whole grains

- healthy fats

The beauty of the diet is that you can still eat many of your favorite (healthy) foods, but only during your eating window. Next, we will look at your eating window options.

Methods in Intermittent Fasting

Intermittent fasting is simply limiting yourself to eating within a designated time frame. There are several variations of IF to choose from. Decide which type fits into your lifestyle the best and then talk about it with your doctor.

Daily method: This is the most popular method of IF. The daily method typically follows a 16/8 or 18/6 rule. That means eating regular, healthy foods during a 6- to 8-hour window each day, then fasting for the remaining 16 to 18 hours. This is found to be the most sustainable method.

You can use other variations of timing to get started. These include a 12/12, which is eating for 12 hours, then fasting for 12 hours. You can then progress to a stricter schedule when you are ready.

5:2 Method: This approach involves eating normal, healthy meals over 5 days of the week and limiting yourself to 500-600 calories during 2 days of the week. It's unclear whether it's more beneficial to eat all your calories in one meal or spread them throughout the day, so do what works for you.

Alternate Day Method: If you choose this method, you can eat normally every other day. On the fasting days, you'll eat just 25% of your daily caloric needs. For example, if you eat 1,800 calories on normal days, you'll only eat 450 calories on the fasting days.

24-Hour Method: This method involves fasting for a full 24 hours before eating again. People who use this method usually fast from breakfast to breakfast or lunch to lunch, and it's usually done only once or twice a week.

Proceed with caution if you use this method. Extreme irritability, fatigue, and headaches can come with it, and this method might not necessarily be better for you.

All the above-mentioned intermittent fasting techniques are proven to be effective as they help lower the blood sugar levels and insulin levels of the body. As a result, women over 50 can kickstart their weight loss through any of these techniques, along with a combination of healthy and nutritious food during the eating hours of the fasting window.

How Does Intermittent Fasting Work

Intermittent fasting simply works by switching between eating and fasting time periods. When the fasting time periods are extended than eating time periods, then your body will burn more calories than usual. Fasting for short time periods is not only helpful for weight loss but also helps in certain health conditions like diabetes, cholesterol, and blood sugar levels.

One thing you need to consider during intermittent fasting; is that what you have been eating. Intermittent fasting works differently for different people. You can adopt any method for intermittent fasting given below:

It might seem strange that simply altering when you eat can help you lose weight. Even so, our bodies respond to fasting in a way that benefits us. When your body enters fasting mode, this triggers your fat stores to be used as fuel, causing you to burn body fat for energy.

Of course, when you are not fasting it doesn't mean you can go crazy with junk food. Stick with nutritious whole foods, unrefined carbohydrates, and lean proteins for the best results. Keep in mind that you can still enjoy calorie-free drinks like black coffee, tea, and water during fasting periods! You might even find yourself slowing down during meals and taking more pleasure in eating.

What Can You Eat When Fasting

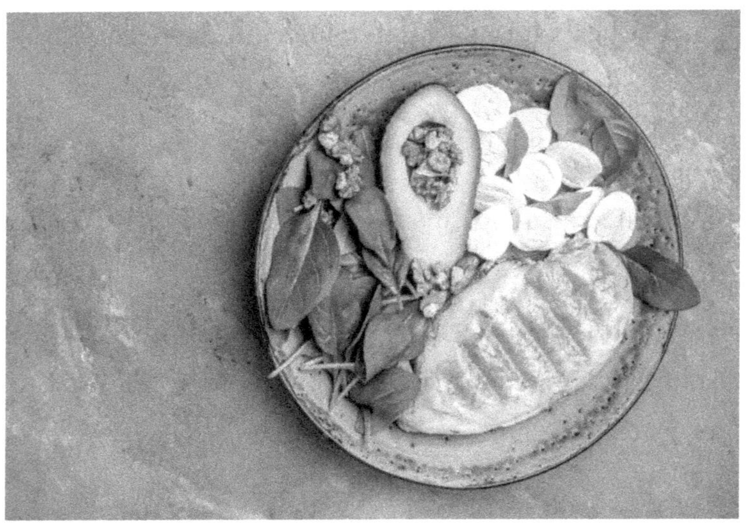

The next question will be what you can eat when fasting to get the best results.

You should not be eating any food during your fasting window, but there are some beverages you can drink that would not break your fast and can even accelerate your results. First and foremost, you make up the bulk of what you consume during your fast.

Coffee and green tea are also excellent choices since they do not contain any calories but contain caffeine and antioxidants. The two of these together can help to accelerate your metabolism, giving you better results than water alone.

Also try mixing in some C8 MCTs to your morning coffee to help fight off the hunger pains while accelerating your metabolism. They're converted into ketones in your body which helps to signal fat burning.

It would be best if you focused on eating quality whole foods and sticking away from processed and refined foods during your feeding window. Inflammatory foods women in their 50s should limit include gluten, dairy, grains, soy, and alcohol, but those will vary depending on the individual.

Eating more protein will be of the essence. You're more likely to experience muscle loss with age, negatively impacting your body composition. Protein also makes you feel fuller longer while helping to build muscle and replace what was lost with age.

Consume your carbohydrates mostly from vegetables and some fruits like berries. Green leafy vegetables like spinach and kale are great choices. Healthy fats like avocados and olive oil should not be avoided since they play a vital role in losing weight and your health.

Women in their 50s will also have a harder time with insulin resistance due to hormonal changes. Therefore, it is best to avoid sugar, starches, and refined carbohydrates.

The trick will be to make sure you are not undereating, which can cause your metabolism to slow and make you feel hungrier, making it harder to fast. Then it becomes easy to overeat the next day out of hunger, putting your hormones and weight fluctuations on a roller coaster.

How Soon Before You See Results From Fasting

One of the many benefits of intermittent fasting is just how fast the results start coming in.

Your weight loss will depend on how much weight you have to lose to begin with. Women who have 30 or more pounds to lose will see the biggest results the fastest. But if you only have 5-10 pounds or so to lose, you will start to see the pounds coming off even after a few days of intermittent fasting.

Intermittent fasting can help promote lean muscle mass, but it is best to add strength training to your workout routine. Muscle and bone loss accelerates for women over 50 so adding in some strength training will help you lose stubborn body fat.

Unfortunately, most make the mistake of just trying to lose weight but need to improve your body composition to tighten up stubborn fat spots.

Once you start losing weight you may experience some loose skin. This is because the collagen in your skin has declined such that it loses elasticity and its ability to snap back. So, adding in strength training can help but it’s also a good idea to take a collagen supplement.

Top Intermittent Fasting Mistakes for Women Over 50

First of all, how is intermittent fasting for women over 50 any different than younger women? Women over 50 tend to have a slower metabolism, may have hormonal imbalances, and may find it more difficult to change their lifestyle. These top intermittent fasting mistakes address some of these differences that affect women over 50.

1. Choosing a Fasting Window That Is Too Short

Women in general benefit from a longer fasting window that is not implemented every single day of the week, but particularly women over 50. Not only will a longer fasting window help ensure that your caloric consumption decreases enough to lose weight (if that is one of your goals), but it will also help you benefit from the metabolic switchover you want.

Ketosis

Switching to fat burning (or ketosis) is what I enjoy most about intermittent fasting. It is what makes it so effective at improving your metabolic health and losing weight.

Most people start exhausting their glycogen stores after fasting for about 12 hours. However, for your body to produce enough ketones to be in ketosis, you most likely need to fast for at least 16-18 hours (unless you eat keto, of course!). Then, you would want to enjoy this metabolic switchover for a while. I tend to recommend a 20-24 hour fast for everyone, but women over 50 will find it even more helpful as they may struggle with insulin resistance.

Alternate-Day Fasting Benefits

Fasting longer and less frequently is an effective option for women over 40. Alternate-day fasting, in particular, has some major benefits. Alternate-day fasting has been shown to increase lifespan in mice. Also, a study where the metabolic effects of fasting were observed at the 12, 36, and 72-hour marks, found that the resting metabolic rate of the subjects increased at 36 hours.

2. Not Cycling Their Diet and Intermittent Fasting Methods

If intermittent fasting for women over 50 involves longer fasts, it also means fewer fasting days. For example, with alternate-day fasting, once or twice a week would be a good goal. If you go for OMAD (One Meal a Day) or the Warrior Diet (fasting for 20 hours), I would recommend you some days off once in a while, particularly before your period.

Again, I want to emphasize that I am not about making rules up. I do want you to be aware of how you feel on your fasting days. After you have gained enough fasting experience, you will know the difference between how you feel on different fasting days. Some days, you will feel hungry but you will be energetic and happy to keep fasting. Some days, you will feel weak and too hungry to fast longer. Listening to your body's cues is an excellent way to cycle your fasting days.

Cycling Your Diet

Similarly, to not always fasting the same length of time every single day of the month, it is a good idea to change things up with your diet. For one thing, it will help you determine which way of eating makes you feel your best, but also, you will notice that your body craves different types of nourishment at different times. Sometimes, eating keto may be just what you need. At other times, you may want to include more carbs in your diet.

3. Not Eating Enough Protein

Again, learning to listen to your body will serve you well in this case. I like to break my fast with the Power Shake because it is light, satisfying, and filled with vitamins and minerals. However, I have noticed that sometimes, I crave meat to break my fast. Those days, I will eat some chicken breast or canned tuna.

As I mentioned, intermittent fasting for women over 50 can be different due to the fact that women over 50 have to deal with a decreasing muscle mass. Increasing your protein intake may help preserve your muscle mass. The recommended protein intake for women is between 10 to 35% of your macronutrients, but as you age, you should aim toward the higher end of that range. Strength training is another effective tool to make sure you stay strong and to mitigate your muscle mass loss. Remember, you can combat muscle loss as you age, but you cannot gain experience unless you age! Let us look at the bright side!

4. Not Drinking Enough Water

It's easy to not drink enough water. You are busy and forget to drink. The first thing you should do any time you feel hungry is drinking a large glass of water. See how you feel after that. Most women need 74 ounces or a bit more than 9 cups of water a day.

Did you know that dehydration is one of the ten most frequent causes of hospitalization for people over 65? I was surprised to learn that! Apparently, as you age, not only does your thirst sensation decrease but your renal water retention as well.

5. Not Dealing With Sleep Issues

Poor sleep is another issue that tends to arise with age. Hormonal changes like the loss of estrogen and progesterone are contributing factors. If you have trouble going to sleep and staying asleep, be aware that there are things you can do to help improve your sleep.

Implementing some sleep habits like going to bed early every night and turning off your screens an hour before bed are obvious ideas. It turns out that exercise is another excellent sleep aid. Make sure you exercise daily (not right before bedtime). Lastly, I have enjoyed a tart cherry concentrate as a means to sleep more soundly. Tart cherries are naturally rich in melatonin, the hormone responsible for good sleep.

Exclusive Tips For You

If you are considering trying intermittent fasting, here are some weight loss tips to help you on your journey:

- Focus on eating bountiful whole foods that stave off hunger and leave you fuller, longer.
- Avoid empty carbs and fast foods, which only temporarily fill you up before the hunger pangs set in.
- Incorporate an exercise routine to help with fat burning and avoid weight gain long-term.
- Experiment with different eating and fasting windows. Your body will respond better to

specific time windows than others, so try a few until you find a rhythm. Women over 50 should start with a 12:12 or 16:8 ratio to allow the body to adjust to this new eating routine.

- Consult with your doctor for medical advice. Your doctor knows your medical history and background and can guide you in approaching intermittent fasting most healthily.
- If you notice weight gain, fatigue, lightheadedness, muscle loss, or insomnia, you might not be getting enough calories. Before you try the diet, use a calorie tracking app like MyFitnessPal to ensure you are getting adequate caloric intake.
- Use this Intermittent Fasting book to stay on track with healthy recipes and tips for daily fasting.

Ready To Give It a Try?

There is a lot to learn about intermittent fasting, but thus far, human studies show that it can promote weight loss and provide abundant health benefits.

However, any time you introduce a new diet or lifestyle choice, it is essential to test the waters. Before going all in, consult with your medical doctor. Also, keep these tips handy to make the transition easier and more sustainable.

CHAPTER TWO

INTERMITTENT FASTING RECIPES

Whether you are eating within a twelve-hour, eight-hour, our four-hour window, you will need substantial go-to meals that will keep you full all day! If you are thinking of consuming a high-protein diet for that very reason, you will find all the options you need right in this chapter.

As is commonly said, breakfast is the most important meal of the day. And this is especially so since it is going to be the meal you break your fast. Here are some nutritious intermittent fasting breakfast recipes you can try out the next time you are in the kitchen.

Breakfast

Poached eggs and bacon on toast

The gentle sizzle of bacon on a pan is the perfect start to anyone's morning. Imagine that meaty, savory smell that lingers in the air even when it's in your stomach; how can anyone get mad after that?

Make your breakfast more filling by topping your toast with eggs, and you never have to worry about a grumbling stomach amid an 11 am meeting again.

Preparation time: 5 minutes

Cooking time: 15 minutes

Makes: 1 toast

INGREDIENTS

- 2 slices bacon
- 2 medium eggs
- 200 grams baby leaf spinach
- Salmon (optional)
- 1 slice of toast
- Sea salt
- Black pepper

DIRECTIONS

- ➢ Bring a large pan of water to a gentle simmer.
- ➢ Swirl the water gently and then crack the eggs in; poach for 4 minutes or until the whites are just set.

- In the meantime, heat a deep-frying pan, add a splash of water and throw in the spinach. Cook for 2 minutes until wilted.
- Remove the spinach and set it aside on a plate. Pan-fry the bacon until golden brown.
- Lay the spinach (and salmon) on the toast, season with salt and pepper.
- Top if all off with the poached eggs and bacon.

Chewy cinnamon rolls (Vegetarian)

There is nothing quite like starting your day off with the welcoming fragrance of cinnamon and freshly baked bread. As implied by its name, these chewy cinnamon rolls are incredibly soft, chewy, and sweet.

Preparation time: 45 minutes, plus an hour and 45 minutes for the dough to rise

Cooking time: 20 minutes

Makes: 24 rolls

INGREDIENTS

Rolls:

- 1 cup whole-wheat flour
- 3 cups all-purpose flour
- ¼ ounce active dry yeast
- 1 cup plain soymilk or milk
- ¾ cup of sugar
- ¼ cup of vegetable oil
- 1 teaspoon salt
- 4 egg whites
- ¼ cup trans-fat-free margarine
- 2 teaspoons cinnamon

Glaze:

- 1 cup powdered sugar
- ½ teaspoon pure vanilla extract
- 2 tablespoons soymilk or milk

DIRECTIONS

- Combine the whole-wheat flour, 1 cup of the all-purpose flour, and the yeast in a large mixing bowl. Set aside.
- Combine the soymilk, ¼ cup of the sugar, the oil, and the salt in a saucepan and heat on low until warm. Stir to blend, and then add to the flour and yeast mixture. Whisk in the egg whites.
- Beat on high speed for about 4 minutes, occasionally stopping to scrape down the sides.
- Stir in most of the remaining all-purpose flour to make a stiff dough.
- Remove the dough from the mixing bowl and set it on a floured surface. Knead the dough for about 10 minutes, adding more flour by the tablespoon as needed to prevent sticking.
- Set the dough in an oiled bowl, and then turn it to oil the top of the dough bowl. Cover with a towel and let it rise in a warm place until doubled in size (roughly an hour).

- Punch the risen dough down and divide it into two pieces. Roll each piece of dough into a rectangle about ¼ inch thick.
- Melt the margarine and brush it onto the rectangle of dough. In a small cup, mix the cinnamon and the remaining ½ cup of sugar, and sprinkle the mixture evenly over both rectangles of dough.
- Roll up the rectangles, starting at the widest ends. Pinch the ends shut with your fingers and press the seams into the dough.
- Cut the rolls into 1-inch pieces, and place the slices cut side down in two oiled baking dishes or 9-inch round non-stick pans. Cover each dish with a towel or waxed paper, and let the rolls rise in a warm place until doubled in size (roughly 45 minutes). Preheat the oven to 375 degrees.
- Bake for 20 minutes.
- While the rolls are baking, prepare the glaze by mixing the confectioner's sugar, vanilla, and 1 tablespoon of the soymilk. Add additional soymilk in increments of 1 teaspoon until the glaze is thick

but pourable. Drizzle the glaze over the warm rolls; enjoy.

Mains

Chilli beef avocado burger

This might be our favorite! Also, if you are concerned about practicing intermittent fasting while on a ketogenic diet, this recipe can be made with skipping the bun; you do not have to give up one for the other. And here is an example of how you can reap both diets' health benefits – in a single dish!

Preparation time: 15 minutes

Cooking time: 10 minutes

Makes: 2 burgers

INGREDIENTS

- 400 grams lean beef mince
- 2 red chilies
- Burger bun (optional)
- Sea salt

- Black pepper
- 1 ripe medium avocado
- 2 sundried tomatoes
- Juice of 1 lemon

DIRECTIONS

- Combine the beef and half of the chopped chilies in a bowl, season with salt and pepper, then divide into four balls. Flatten each into a thin patty and set aside.
- Halve the avocados, scoop the flesh into a bowl and mash with a fork.
- Stir in the remaining chili, the sundried tomatoes, and the lemon juice with the mashed avocados.
- Put a tablespoon of the avocado mixture in the center of the two patties, then top each with the remaining patties. Press down the edges to seal the avocado in the middle of the burger.
- Heat a griddle pan to high heat, add the burgers, and cook for 5 minutes on each side until cooked through.

- If you decide to use buns, simply put the cooked avocado patties between two buns (you can use only one if you want to reduce the number of calories). To make yourself feel satiated for longer, consider using a full-grain bun option.

Cajun red beans and rice (Vegetarian)

If the thought of spending hours in the kitchen terrifies you, you will appreciate the fuss-free nature of this dish. So long as you make the rice ahead of time, you will find that this American, south-coastal traditional dish takes very little time to prepare.

Preparation time: 10 minutes

Cooking time: 15 minutes

Makes: 8 servings

INGREDIENTS

- 3 tablespoons olive oil
- 1 large onion, chopped
- 3 cloves garlic, minced

- ½ cup chopped green bell pepper
- 1 stalk celery, including green leaves, chopped
- ½ teaspoon salt
- 1 teaspoon cumin
- 1 tablespoon chili powder
- ½ teaspoon thyme
- Two 15-ounce cans dark red kidney beans, rinsed and drained
- 20½ cups cooked rice
- Fresh parsley for garnish

DIRECTIONS

- ➢ Heat the olive oil in a large skillet. Cook the onions, garlic, bell pepper, and celery in the oil over medium heat until the onions are translucent (roughly 7 minutes). Add the salt, cumin, chili powder, and thyme. Stir to combine.
- ➢ Add the beans and mix well. Reduce the heat to low and continue cooking for several minutes until the beans are hot. Be sure to stir frequently to prevent sticking.

- ➢ Add the rice to the bean mixture and mix all the ingredients well. Cook for about 5 minutes to heat the rice through before serving.
- ➢ Garnish with sprigs of parsley and Enjoy!

Other go-to meal are:

Spicy Chocolate Keto Fat Bombs

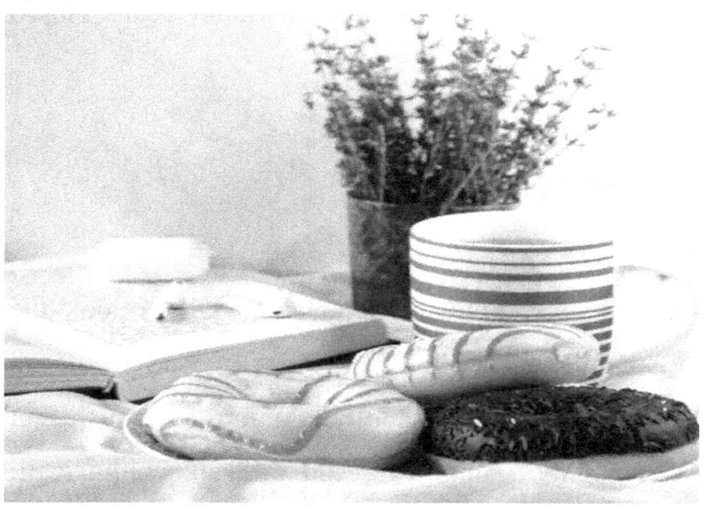

Preparation Time: 10 minutes

INGREDIENTS

- 2⁄3 cup coconut oil
- 2⁄3 cup smooth peanut butter

- 1⁄2 cup dark cocoa
- 4 (6 g) packets stevia (or to taste)
- 1 tablespoon ground cinnamon
- 1⁄4 teaspoon kosher salt
- 1⁄2 cup toasted coconut flakes
- 1⁄4 teaspoon cayenne (to taste)

DIRECTIONS

- Combine coconut oil, peanut butter, and cocoa powder in a double boiler set over a pot of simmering water. Heat, whisking, until melted and smooth.
- Add stevia, cinnamon, and salt and stir to combine.
- Divide mixture among a silicone mini muffin tray. (Alternatively, line a mini muffin tin with liners and divide mixture among liners.).
- Top with coconut and cayenne and transfer to freezer until firm, about 30 minutes.

NUTRITION INFO

Serving Size: 1 (17) g

Servings Per Recipe: 24

AMT. PER SERVING	% DAILY VALUE
Calories: 110	
Calories from Fat 93 g	85%
Total Fat 10.3 g	15%
Saturated Fat 6.5 g	32%
Cholesterol 0 mg	0%
Sodium 62.2 mg	2%
Total Carbohydrate 3.6 g	1%
Dietary Fiber 1.1 g	4%
Sugars 1.3 g	5%
Protein 2.2 g	4%

Grilled Lemon Salmon

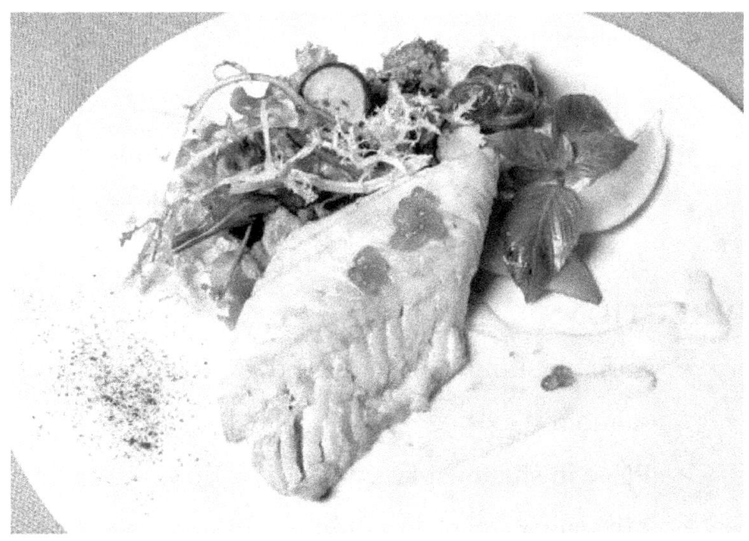

Preparation Time: 30 minutes

INGREDIENTS

- 2 teaspoons fresh dill
- 1⁄2 teaspoon pepper
- 1⁄2 teaspoon salt
- 1⁄2 teaspoon garlic powder
- 1 1⁄2 lbs salmon fillets
- 1⁄4 cup packed brown sugar
- 1 chicken bouillon cube, mixed with

- 3 tablespoons water
- 3 tablespoons oil
- 3 tablespoons soy sauce
- 4 tablespoons finely chopped green onions
- 1 lemon, thinly sliced
- 2 slices onions, separated into rings

DIRECTIONS

- Sprinkle dill, pepper, salt and garlic powder over salmon.
- Place in shallow glass pan.
- Mix sugar, chicken bouillon, oil, soy sauce, and green onions.
- Pour over salmon.
- Cover and chill for 1 hour, turn once.
- Drain and discard marinade.
- Put on grill on med heat, place lemon and onion on top.
- Cover and cook for 15 minutes, or until fish is done.

NUTRITION INFO

Serving Size: 1 (249) g

Servings Per Recipe: 4

AMT. PER SERVING	% DAILY VALUE
Calories: 380.7	
Calories from Fat 161 g	42 %
Total Fat 17.9 g	27%
Saturated Fat 2.8 g	13%
Cholesterol 78.6 mg	26%
Sodium 1417.5 mg	59%
Total Carbohydrate 17.3g	5%
Dietary Fiber 0.9 g	3%
Sugars 14.6 g	58%
Protein 37 g	74%

Avocado Quesadillas

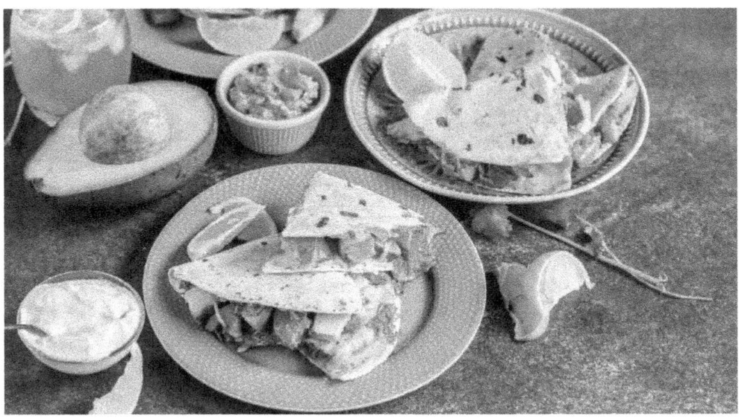

Preparation Time: 35 minutes

INGREDIENTS

- 2 vine-ripe tomatoes, seeded and chopped into 1/4 inch pieces
- 1 ripe avocado, peeled, pitted, and chopped into 1/4 inch pieces
- 1 tablespoon chopped red onion
- 2 teaspoons fresh lemon juice
- 1⁄4 teaspoon Tabasco sauce
- salt and pepper
- 1⁄4 cup sour cream
- 3 tablespoons chopped fresh coriander
- 24 inches flour tortillas
- 1⁄2 teaspoon vegetable oil
- 1 1⁄3 cups shredded monterey jack cheese

DIRECTIONS

- In a small bowl, mix together the tomatoes, avocado, onion, lemon juice and Tabasco.
- Season to taste with salt and pepper.

- In another small bowl, mix together sour cream, coriander, salt and pepper to taste.
- Put tortillas on a baking sheet and brush tops with oil.
- Broil tortillas 2 to 4 inches from heat until pale golden.
- Sprinkle tortillas evenly with cheese and broil until cheese is melted.
- Spread avocado mixture evenly over 2 tortillas and top each with 1 of remaining tortillas, cheese side down to make 2 quesadillas.
- Transfer quesadillas to a cutting board and cut into 4 wedges.
- Top each wedge with a dollop of sour cream mixture and serve warm.

NUTRITION INFO

Serving Size: 1 (425) g

Servings Per Recipe: 2

AMT. PER SERVING	% DAILY VALUE
Calories: 794.9	
Calories from Fat 460 g	58%
Total Fat 51.1 g	78%
Saturated Fat 21.6 g	107%
Cholesterol 82 mg	27%
Sodium 978.8 mg	40%
Total Carbohydrate 58.7 g	19%
Dietary Fiber 11 g	23%
Sugars 7.2 g	28%
Protein 29.2 g	58%

Veggie-Packed Cheesy Chicken Salad

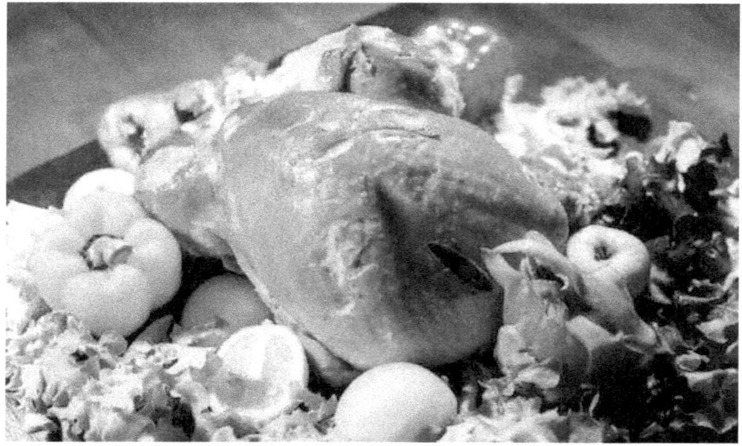

Preparation Time: 34 minutes

INGREDIENTS

- 1 cup cooked boneless skinless chicken breast, cubed
- 1⁄4 cup celery, finely chopped
- 1⁄4 cup carrot, shaved into ribbons
- 1⁄2 cup Baby Spinach, roughly chopped
- 2 1⁄2 tablespoons fat-free mayonnaise
- 2 tablespoons nonfat sour cream
- 1⁄8 teaspoon dried parsley
- 2 teaspoons Dijon mustard
- 1⁄4 cup reduced-fat sharp cheddar cheese, shredded

DIRECTIONS

- Mix all ingredients in a bowl so that everything is coated well with the mayonnaise mixture.
- Chill in the fridge for at least 30 minutes but you could do it the night before.
- Serve.

NUTRITION INFO

Serving Size: 1 (161) g

Servings Per Recipe: 1

AMT. PER SERVING	% DAILY VALUE
Calories: 364.5	
Calories from Fat 81 g	22%
Total Fat 9.1 g	13%
Saturated Fat 3.1 g	15%
Cholesterol 131.8 mg	43%
Sodium 767.4 mg	31%
Total Carbohydrate 15.3 g	5%
Dietary Fiber 2.8 g	11%
Sugars 7.3 g	29%
Protein 53.2 g	106%

Cobb Salad With Brown Derby Dressing

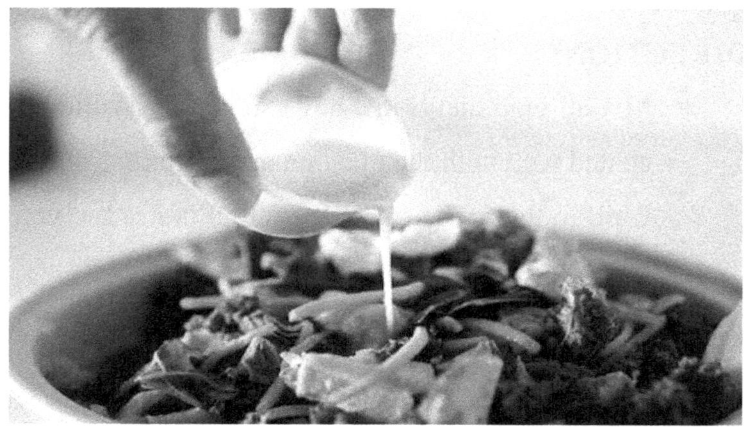

Preparation Time: 32 minutes

INGREDIENTS

- 1⁄2 head iceberg lettuce
- 1⁄2 bunch watercress
- 1 bunch chicory lettuce
- 1⁄2 head romaine lettuce
- 2 medium tomatoes, skinned and seeded
- 1⁄2 lb smoked turkey breast
- 6 slices crisp bacon
- 1 avocado, sliced in half,seeded and peeled
- 3 hardboiled egg
- 2 tablespoons chives, chopped fine
- 1⁄2 cup blue cheese, crumbled

DRESSING

- 2 tablespoons water
- 1⁄8 teaspoon sugar
- 3⁄4 teaspoon kosher salt
- 1⁄2 teaspoon Worcestershire sauce
- 2 tablespoons balsamic vinegar (or red wine vinegar)

- 1 tablespoon fresh lemon juice
- 1⁄2 teaspoon fresh ground black pepper
- 1⁄8 teaspoon Dijon mustard
- 2 tablespoons olive oil
- 2 cloves garlic, minced very fine

DIRECTIONS

- ➢ Chop all the greens very, very fine (almost minced).
- ➢ Arrange in rows in a chilled salad bowl.
- ➢ Cut the tomatoes in half, seed, and chop very fine.
- ➢ Fine dice the turkey, avocado, eggs and bacon.
- ➢ Arrange all the ingredients, including the blue cheese, in rows across the lettuces.
- ➢ Sprinkle with the chives.
- ➢ Present at the table in this fashion, then toss with the dressing at the very last minute and serve in chilled salad bowls.
- ➢ Serve with fresh french bread.

FOR THE DRESSING:

- Combine all the ingredients except the olive oil in a blender and blend.
- Slowly, with the machine running, add the oil and blend well.
- Keep refrigerated.

NOTE: This dish should be kept chilled, and served as chilled as possible.

NUTRITION INFO

Serving Size: 1 (821) g

Servings Per Recipe: 2

AMT. PER SERVING	% DAILY VALUE
Calories: 832.4	
Calories from Fat 510 g	61%
Total Fat 56.7 g	87%
Saturated Fat 16.1 g	80%
Cholesterol 352.4 mg	117%
Sodium 3360.1 mg	140%
Total Carbohydrate 31.2 g	10%
Dietary Fiber 13.5 g	53%
Sugars 12.4 g	49%
Protein 55 g	109%

Vegan Fried 'Fish' Tacos

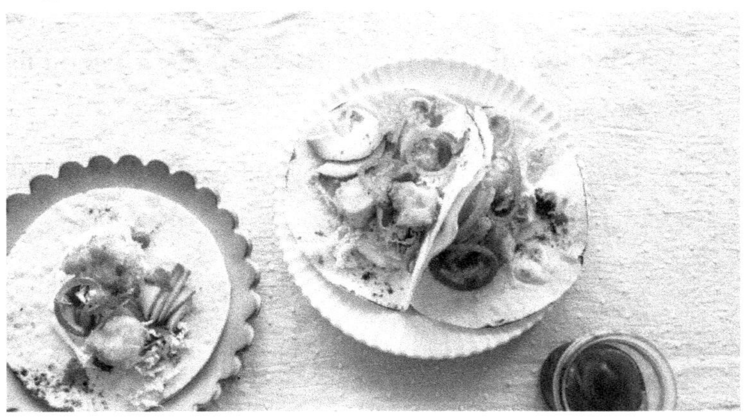

Preparation Time: 55 minutes

INGREDIENTS

- 14 ounces silken tofu
- 2 cups panko breadcrumbs
- 1⁄2 cup plain flour
- 1⁄2 teaspoon salt
- 1 teaspoon smoked paprika
- 1⁄2 teaspoon cayenne pepper
- 1 teaspoon ground cumin
- 1⁄2 cup non-dairy milk

- vegetable oil, for frying
- 1⁄4 head cabbage, finely shredded
- 1 ripe avocado
- 8 small tortillas
- vegan mayonnaise, to serve

PICKLED ONION

- 1 red onion, peeled, finely sliced
- 1⁄4 cup apple cider vinegar
- 1 tablespoon sugar
- 1 teaspoon salt

DIRECTIONS

- ➢ Pat the tofu with a few pieces of kitchen roll to remove excess moisture. Use a knife to break the tofu into rough 1-inch chunks – I like them to be imperfect, not cubes, so they look nicer!
- ➢ Place the breadcrumbs into one wide shallow bowl.
- ➢ Place the flour, salt, smoked paprika, cayenne and cumin into another wide shallow bowl and stir together.
- ➢ Place the milk into a third wide shallow bowl.

- Take the chunks of tofu and gently coat them in the flour then the milk then the breadcrumbs and onto a baking sheet.
- Fill a deep frying pan with 1/2 -inch depth of vegetable oil. Place over a medium heat and let the oil get hot – sprinkle a breadcrumb in and if it start to bubble and brown, the oil is hot enough. Add chunks of breaded tofu to the oil and fry until golden underneath then flip and cook so it’s golden all over. Remove to a baking sheet lined with kitchen roll to drain. Repeat with the remaining tofu.

FOR THE PICKLED ONION:

- Heat the apple cide vinegar, salt and sugar in a small pot until steaming. Place the finely sliced red onion in a bowl or jar and pour the hot vinegar over. Let it sit for at least 30 minutes to soften and turn pink.
- Serve the hot fried tofu in warmed tortillas (I warm them over the lit gas ring of my stove), pickled

onion, a smear of vegan mayo, some avocado and shredded cabbage.

Mediterranean Chicken Breasts With Avocado Tapenade

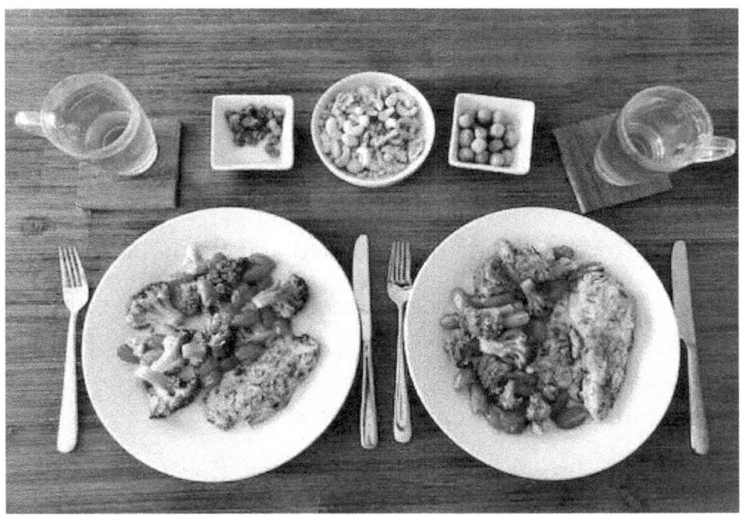

Preparation Time: 17 minutes

INGREDIENTS

- 4 boneless skinless chicken breast halves
- 1 tablespoon grated lemon peel
- 5 tablespoons fresh lemon juice, divided

- 2 tablespoons olive oil, divided
- 1 teaspoon olive oil, divided
- 1 garlic clove, finely chopped
- 1/2 teaspoon salt
- 1/4 teaspoon ground black pepper
- 2 garlic cloves, roasted and mashed
- 1/2 teaspoon sea salt
- 1/4 teaspoon fresh ground pepper
- 1 medium tomatoes, seeded and finely chopped
- 1/4 cup small green pimento stuffed olive, thinly sliced
- 3 tablespoons capers, rinsed
- 2 tablespoons fresh basil leaves, finely sliced
- 1 large Hass avocado, ripe, finely chopped

DIRECTIONS

- In sealable plastic bag, combine chicken and marinade of lemon peel, 2 tablespoons lemon juice, 2 tablespoons olive oil, garlic, salt and pepper. Seal bag and refrigerate for 30 minutes.

- In bowl, whisk together remaining 3 tablespoons lemon juice, roasted garlic, remaining 1/2 teaspoons olive oil, sea salt and fresh ground pepper. Mix in tomato, green olives, capers, basil and avocado; set aside.
- Remove chicken from bag and discard marinade. Grill over medium-hot coals for 4 to 5 minutes per side or to desired degree of doneness.
- Serve with Avocado Tapenade.

NUTRITION INFO

Serving Size: 1 (222) g

Servings Per Recipe: 4

AMT. PER SERVING	% DAILY VALUE
Calories: 277.1	
Calories from Fat 147 g	61%
Total Fat 16.4 g	87%
Saturated Fat 2.5 g	80%
Cholesterol 75.5 mg	117%
Sodium 914.6 mg	140%
Total Carbohydrate 6.9 g	10%
Dietary Fiber 3.2 g	53%
Sugars 1.5 g	49%
Protein 26.4 g	109%

Supper Club Tilapia Parmesan

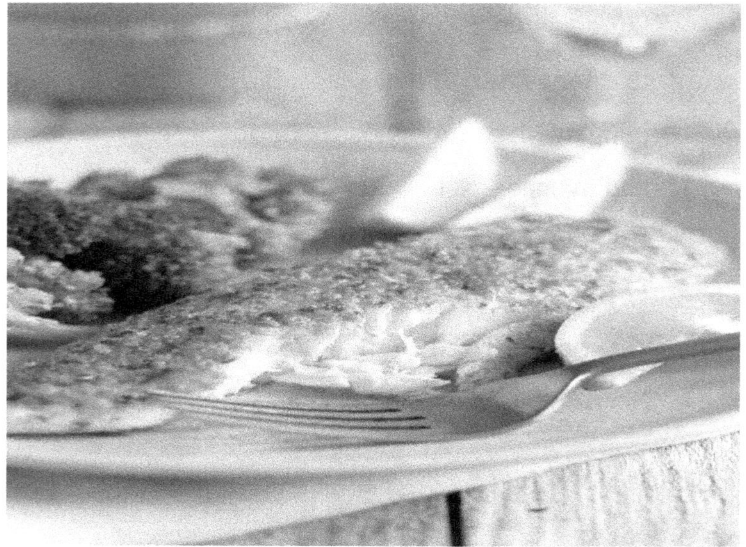

Preparation Time: 35 minutes

INGREDIENTS

- 2 lbs tilapia fillets (orange roughie, cod or red snapper can be substituted)
- 2 tablespoons lemon juice
- 1⁄2 cup grated parmesan cheese
- 4 tablespoons butter, room temperature
- 3 tablespoons mayonnaise
- 3 tablespoons finely chopped green onions

- 1/4 teaspoon seasoning salt
- 1/4 teaspoon dried basil
- black pepper
- 1 dash hot pepper sauce

DIRECTIONS

- Preheat oven to 350 degrees.
- In buttered 13-by-9-inch baking dish or jellyroll pan, lay fillets in single layer.
- Do not stack fillets.
- Brush top with juice.
- In bowl combine cheese, butter, mayonnaise, onions and seasonings.
- Mix well with fork.
- Bake fish in preheated oven 10 to 20 minutes or until fish just starts to flake.
- Spread with cheese mixture and bake until golden brown, about 5 minutes.
- Baking time will depend on the thickness of the fish you use.
- Watch fish closely so that it does not overcook.
- Makes 4 servings.

Note: This fish can also be made in a broiler.

- Broil 3 to 4 minutes or until almost done.
- Add cheese and broil another 2 to 3 minutes or until browned.

NUTRITION INFO

Serving Size: 1 (266) g

Servings Per Recipe: 4

AMT. PER SERVING	% DAILY VALUE
Calories: 376.8	
Calories from Fat 170 g	45%
Total Fat 19 g	29%
Saturated Fat 10.8 g	53%
Cholesterol 155 mg	51%
Sodium 413.3 mg	17%
Total Carbohydrate 1.4 g	0%
Dietary Fiber 0.2 g	0%
Sugars 0.4 g	1%
Protein 50.6 g	101%

Shredded Brussels Sprouts With Bacon & Onions

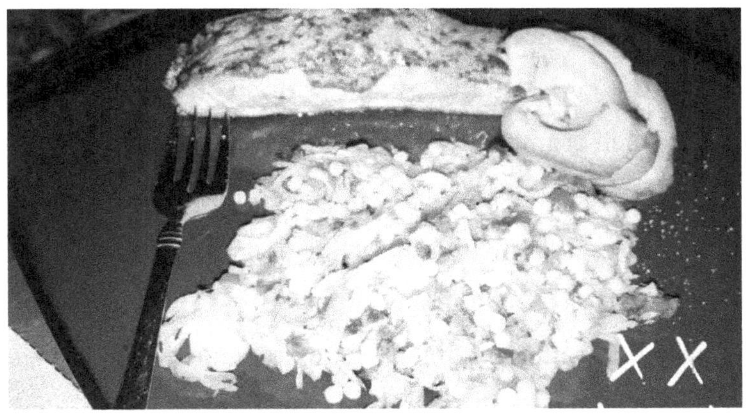

Preparation Time: 32 minutes

INGREDIENTS

- 2 slices bacon
- 1 small yellow onion, thinly sliced
- 1⁄4 teaspoon salt (or to taste)
- 3⁄4 cup water
- 1 teaspoon Dijon mustard
- 1 lb Brussels sprout, trimmed, halved and very thinly sliced
- 1 tablespoon cider vinegar

DIRECTIONS

- Cook bacon in a large skillet over medium heat until crisp (5 to 7 minutes); drain on paper towels, then crumble.
- Add onion and salt to the drippings in the pan and cook over medium heat, stirring often, until tender and browned (about 3 minutes).
- Add water and mustard, scraping up any browned bits, then add Brussels sprouts and cook, stirring often, until tender (4 to 6 minutes).
- Stir in vinegar and top with the crumbled bacon.

NUTRITION INFO

Serving Size: 1 (123) g

Servings Per Recipe: 6

AMT. PER SERVING	% DAILY VALUE
Calories: 45.2	
Calories from Fat 14 g	32%
Total Fat 1.6 g	2%
Saturated Fat 0.5 g	2%
Cholesterol 1.8 mg	0%
Sodium 145.9 mg	6%
Total Carbohydrate 6.5 g	2%
Dietary Fiber 2.2 g	8%
Sugars 1.8 g	7%
Protein 2.4 g	4%

Cauliflower Popcorn

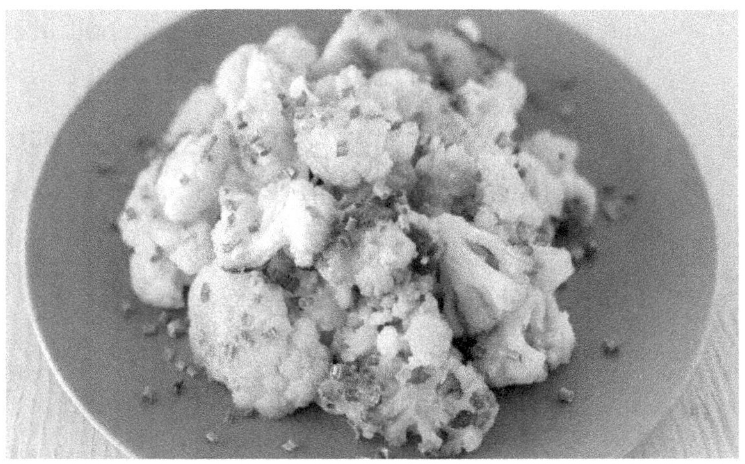

Preparation Time: 65 minutes

INGREDIENTS

- 1 head cauliflower or 1 head equal amount of pre-cut commercially prepped cauliflower
- 4 tablespoons olive oil
- 1 teaspoon salt, to taste

DIRECTIONS

- Preheat oven to 425 degrees.

- Trim the head of cauliflower, discarding the core and thick stems; cut florets into pieces about the size of ping-pong balls.
- In a large bowl, combine the olive oil and salt, whisk, then add the cauliflower pieces and toss thoroughly.
- Line a baking sheet with parchment for easy cleanup (you can skip that, if you don't have any) then spread the cauliflower pieces on the sheet and roast for 1 hour, turning 3 or 4 times, until most of each piece has turned golden brown.
- (The browner the cauliflower pieces turn, the more caramelization occurs and the sweeter they will taste).
- Serve immediately and enjoy!

NUTRITION INFO

Serving Size: 1 (162) g

Servings Per Recipe: 4

AMT. PER SERVING	% DAILY VALUE
Calories: 156.1	
Calories from Fat 125 g	80%
Total Fat 13.9 g	21%
Saturated Fat 2 g	9%
Cholesterol 0 mg	0%
Sodium 625.7 mg	26%
Total Carbohydrate 7.3 g	2%
Dietary Fiber 2.9 g	11%
Sugars 2.8 g	11%
Protein 2.8 g	5%

Baked Potato

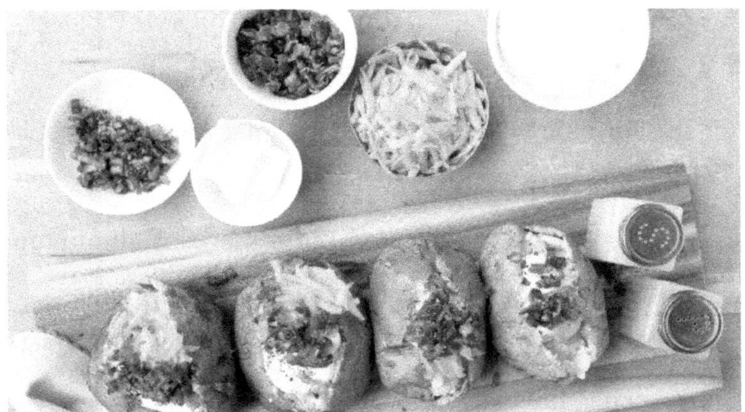

Preparation Time: 70 minutes

INGREDIENTS

- 1 large russet potato
- canola oil
- kosher salt

DIRECTIONS

- Heat oven to 350°F and position racks in top and bottom thirds.
- Wash potato (or potatoes) thoroughly with a stiff brush and cold running water.
- Dry, then using a standard fork poke 8 to 12 deep holes all over the spud so that moisture can escape during cooking.
- Place in a bowl and coat lightly with oil.
- Sprinkle with kosher salt and place potato directly on rack in middle of oven.
- Place a baking sheet (I put a piece of aluminum foil) on the lower rack to catch any drippings.
- Bake 1 hour or until skin feels crisp but flesh beneath feels soft.

- Serve by creating a dotted line from end to end with your fork, then crack the spud open by squeezing the ends towards one another.
- It will pop right open.
- But watch out, there will be some steam.

NOTE: If you are cooking more than 4 potatoes, you will need to extend the cooking time by up to 15 minutes.

NUTRITION INFO

Serving Size: 1 (369) g

Servings Per Recipe: 1

AMT. PER SERVING	% DAILY VALUE
Calories: 284.1	
Calories from Fat 2 g	1%
Total Fat 0.3 g	0%
Saturated Fat 0.1 g	0%
Cholesterol 0 mg	0%
Sodium 22.1 mg	0%
Total Carbohydrate 64.5 g	21%
Dietary Fiber 8.1 g	32%
Sugars 2.9 g	11%
Protein 7.5 g	14%

Black Bean Soup

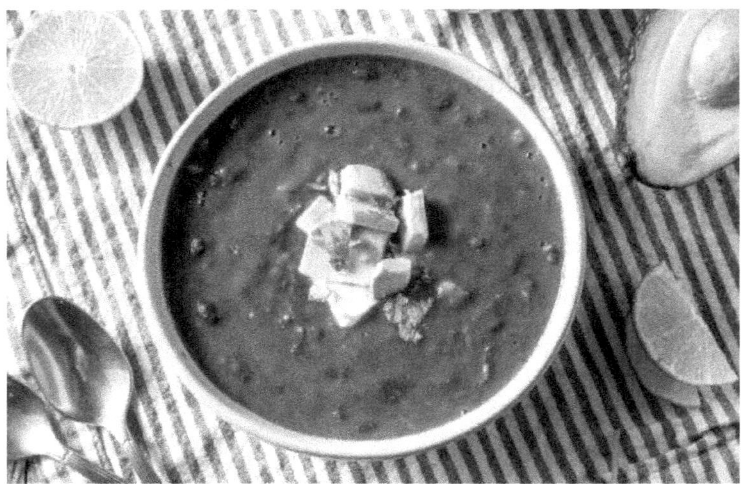

Preparation Time: 22 minutes

INGREDIENTS

- 3 tablespoons olive oil
- 1 medium onion, chopped
- 1 tablespoon ground cumin
- 2 -3 cloves garlic
- 2 (14 1/2 ounce) cans black beans
- 2 cups chicken broth or 2 cups vegetable broth
- salt and pepper

- 1 small red onion, chopped fine
- 1⁄4 cup cilantro, coarsely chopped or finely chopped (whatever you prefer)

DIRECTIONS

- Saute onion in olive oil.
- When onion becomes translucent, add cumin.
- Cook 30 seconds, then add garlic and cook for another 30 to 60 seconds.
- Add 1 can black beans and 2 cups vegetable broth.
- Bring to a simmer, stirring occasionally.
- Turn off heat.
- Using a hand blender, blend the ingredients in the pot, or transfer to a blender.
- Add the second can of beans to the pot along with blended ingredients and bring to a simmer.
- Serve soup with bowls of red onion and cilantro for garnish.

NUTRITION INFO

Serving Size: 1 (329) g

Servings Per Recipe: 4

AMT. PER SERVING	% DAILY VALUE
Calories: 331.1	
Calories from Fat 108 g	33%
Total Fat 12 g	18%
Saturated Fat 1.8 g	9%
Cholesterol 0 mg	0%
Sodium 380 mg	15%
Total Carbohydrate 41.1 g	13%
Dietary Fiber 13.9 g	55%
Sugars 2.3 g	9%
Protein 16.5 g	33%

Vegan Lentil Burgers

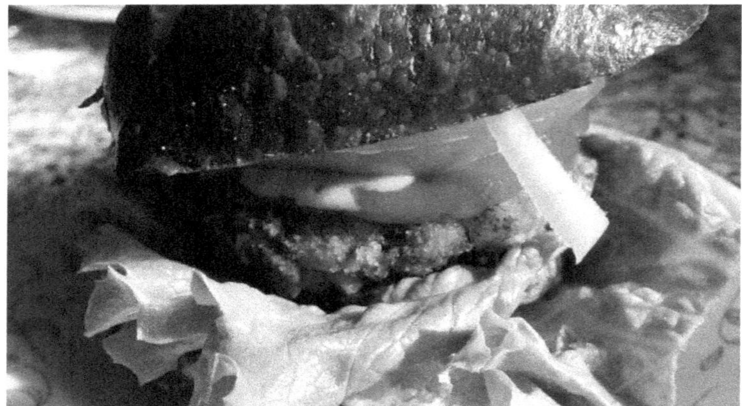

Preparation Time: 65 minutes

INGREDIENTS

1 cup dry lentils, well rinsed

2 1⁄2 cups water

1⁄2 teaspoon salt

1 tablespoon olive oil

1⁄2 medium onion, diced

1 carrot, diced

1 teaspoon pepper

1 tablespoon soy sauce

3⁄4 cup rolled oats, finely ground

3⁄4 cup breadcrumbs

DIRECTIONS

- Boil lentils in the water with the salt for around 45 minutes. Lentils will be soft and most of the water will be gone.
- Fry the onions and carrot in the oil until soft, it will take about 5 minutes.
- In a bowl mix the cooked ingredients with the pepper, soy sauce, oats and bread cumbs.

- While still warm form the mixture into patties, it will make 8-10 burgers.
- Burgers can then be shallow fried for 1-2 minutes on each side or baked at 200C for 15 minutes.

NUTRITION INFO

Serving Size: 1 (1079) g

Servings Per Recipe: 1

AMT. PER SERVING	% DAILY VALUE
Calories: 176.4	
Calories from Fat 27 g	15%
Total Fat 3 g	4%
Saturated Fat 0.5 g	2%
Cholesterol 0 mg	0%
Sodium 354.9 mg	14%
Total Carbohydrate 28.5 g	9%
Dietary Fiber 9 g	35%
Sugars 1.9 g	7%
Protein 9g	17%

Sauerkraut Salad

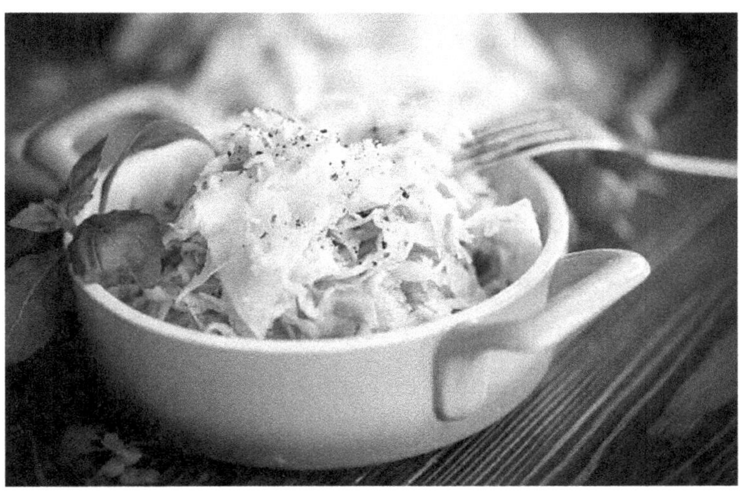

Preparation Time: 12 minutes

INGREDIENTS

- 1 (1 lb) can sauerkraut, drained but not rinsed
- 1 cup celery, chopped fine
- 1/2 cup green pepper, chopped fine
- 2 tablespoons onions, chopped fine
- 1/2 teaspoon salt
- 1/2 teaspoon pepper
- 3/4 cup sugar

- 1⁄3 cup salad oil
- 1⁄3 cup cider or 1/3 cup white vinegar (I use white)

DIRECTIONS

- Mix chopped vegetables with sauerkraut.
- Heat sugar, oil, vinegar, salt, and pepper over low heat just until sugar dissolves.
- Cool and pour over vegetables.
- Chill overnight.

NUTRITION INFO

Serving Size: 1 (145) g

Servings Per Recipe: 6

AMT. PER SERVING	% DAILY VALUE
Calories: 224.1	
Calories from Fat 109 g	49%
Total Fat 12.2 g	18%
Saturated Fat 1.7 g	8%
Cholesterol 0 mg	0%
Sodium 708.5 mg	29%
Total Carbohydrate 29.7 g	9%
Dietary Fiber 2.8 g	11%
Sugars 27.1 g	108%
Protein 1 g	1%

Weight Watchers Berry Crisp

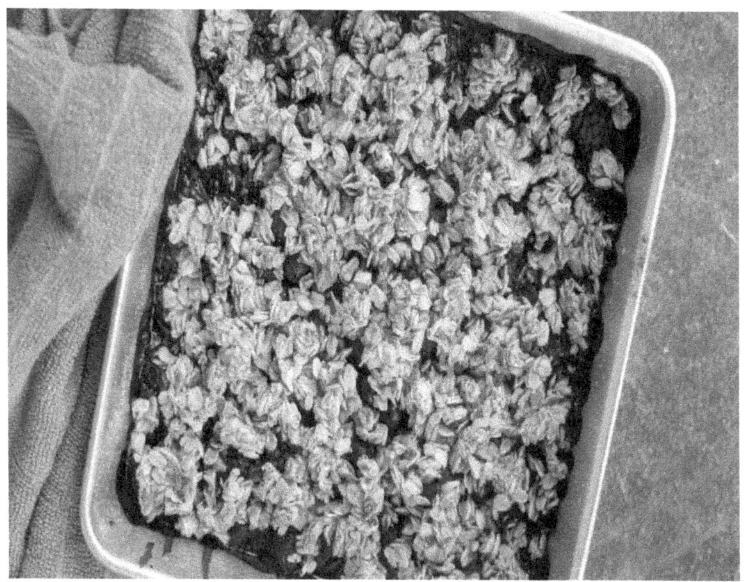

Preparation Time: 40 minutes

INGREDIENTS

FRUIT

- 1 (16 ounce) bag cherries or (16 ounce) bag blueberries
- 1 (7/8 ounce) box jello sugar-free vanilla pudding mix, cook and serve
- 1 teaspoon cinnamon

- 1⁄2 teaspoon nutmeg
- 1⁄4 cup nonfat milk

CRISP

- 1 1⁄2 cups old fashioned oats
- 1⁄2 cup Splenda sugar substitute
- 8 ounces plain fat-free yogurt
- 1 teaspoon almond extract

DIRECTIONS

- Spray an 8X8 baking pan.
- Mix the fruit ingredients in the pan and stir well.
- In a separate bowl, mix together crisp mix.
- Spread this mixture over the berry mixture to make a top crust.
- Bake at 350°F for 40-45 minutes or until topping gets crunchy.

NUTRITION INFO

Serving Size: 1 (74) g

Servings Per Recipe: 6

AMT. PER SERVING	% DAILY VALUE
Calories: 121.6	
Calories from Fat 13 g	11%
Total Fat 1.5 g	2%
Saturated Fat 0.3 g	1%
Cholesterol 1 mg	0%
Sodium 34.6 mg	1%
Total Carbohydrate 22 g	7%
Dietary Fiber 2.2 g	9%
Sugars 7.6 g	30%
Protein 5.2 g	10%

Baked Mahi Mahi

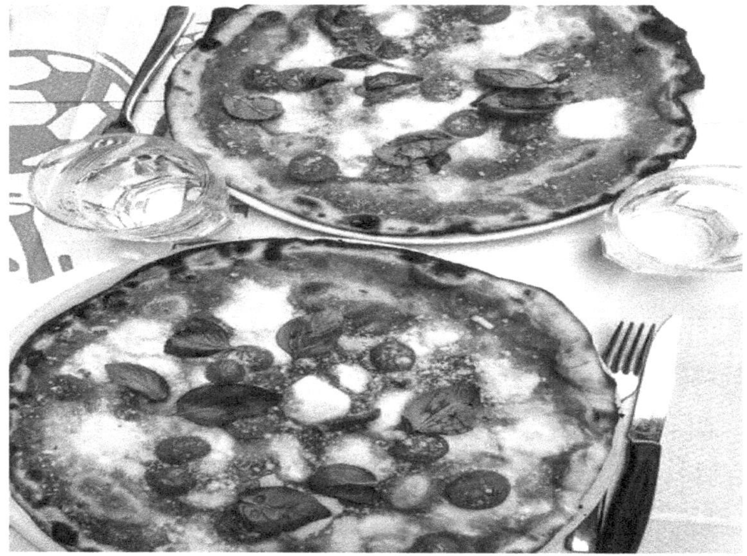

Preparation Time: 35 minutes

INGREDIENTS

- 2 lbs mahi mahi (4 fillets)
- 1 lemon, juiced
- 1⁄4 teaspoon garlic salt
- 1⁄4 teaspoon ground black pepper
- 1 cup mayonnaise
- 1⁄4 cup white onion, finely chopped breadcrumbs

DIRECTIONS

- Preheat oven to 425°F.
- Rinse fish and put in a baking dish. Squeeze lemon juice on fish then sprinkle with garlic salt and pepper.
- Mix mayonnaise and chopped onions and spread on fish. Sprinkle with breadcrumbs and bake at 425°F for 25 minutes.

NUTRITION INFO

Serving Size: 1 (251) g

Servings Per Recipe: 4

AMT. PER SERVING	% DAILY VALUE
Calories: 201.9	
Calories from Fat 14 g	7%
Total Fat 1.6 g	2%
Saturated Fat 0.4 g	2%
Cholesterol 165.5 mg	55%
Sodium 200.3 mg	8%
Total Carbohydrate 2.5 g	0%
Dietary Fiber 0.6 g	2%
Sugars 0.8 g	3%
Protein 42.2 g	84%

Broccoli Dal Curry

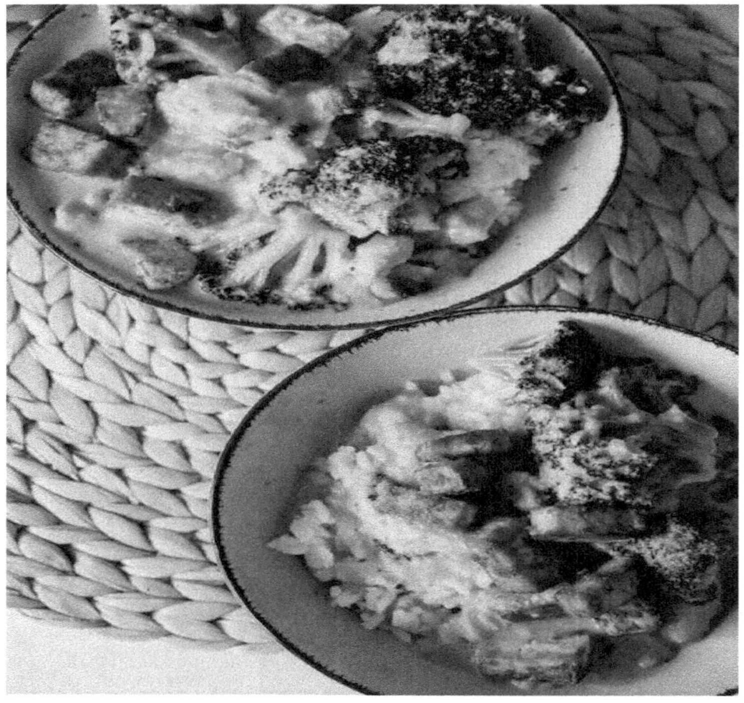

Wow, so easy and delicious. It is double-helping awesome! I served it without rice. It is so gratifying to find a staple like this. I could make a big batch and eat from it all week long.

Preparation Time: 80 minutes

INGREDIENTS

- 4 tablespoons butter or 4 tablespoons ghee
- 2 medium onions, chopped
- 1 teaspoon chili powder
- 1 1⁄2 teaspoons black pepper
- 2 teaspoons cumin
- 1 teaspoon ground coriander
- 2 teaspoons turmeric
- 1 cup red lentil
- 1 lemon, juice of
- 3 cups chicken broth
- 2 medium broccoli, chopped
- 1⁄2 cup dried coconut (optional)
- 1 tablespoon flour
- 1 teaspoon salt
- 1 cup cashews, coarsely chopped (optional)

DIRECTIONS

- Heat butter in saucepan and sate onions until well browned.

- Add chili powder, pepper, cumin, coriander and turmeric.
- Stir and cook, 1 minute.
- Add lentils, lemon juice, broth and coconut if using.
- Bring to boil, reduce heat and simmer for 45-55 minutes (if mixture is too thick, you may need to add a little hot water).
- Steam broccoli for 7 minutes.
- Plunge broccoli in cold water and set aside.
- Remove 1/3 cup of liquid from the lentil mixture.
- Add to flour to form a smooth paste.
- Return to pan; add broccoli, salt and nuts if using.
- Simmer for 5 minutes.
- Serve over Basmati rice.

NUTRITION INFO

Serving Size: 1 (669) g

Servings Per Recipe: 4

AMT. PER SERVING	% DAILY VALUE
Calories: 445	
Calories from Fat 138 g	31%
Total Fat 15.4 g	23%
Saturated Fat 8 g	40%
Cholesterol 30.5 mg	10%
Sodium 1362.4 mg	56%
Total Carbohydrate 59 g	19%
Dietary Fiber 15.1 g	60%
Sugars 8.5 g	33%
Protein 25.7 g	51%

Sweet Potato & Black Bean Burrito

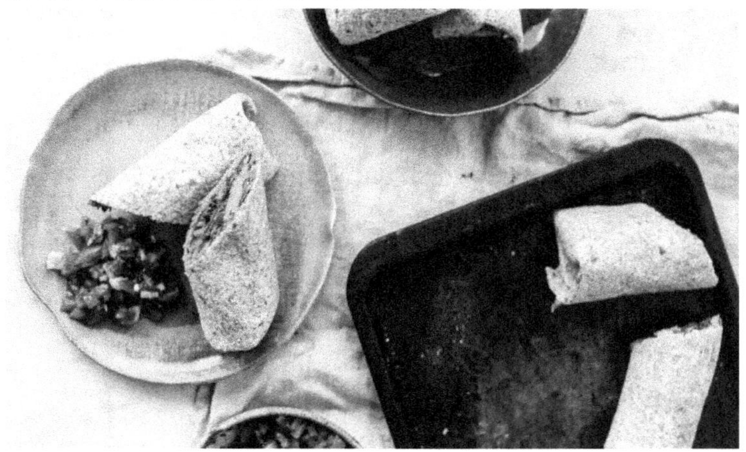

Preparation Time: 60 minutes

INGREDIENTS

- 5 cups peeled cubed sweet potatoes
- 1⁄2 teaspoon salt
- 2 teaspoons other vegetable oil or 2 teaspoons broth
- 3 1⁄2 cups diced onions
- 4 garlic cloves, minced (or pressed)
- 1 tablespoon minced fresh green chili pepper
- 4 teaspoons ground cumin
- 4 teaspoons ground coriander
- 4 1⁄2 cups cooked black beans (three 15-ounce cans, drained)
- 2⁄3 cup lightly packed cilantro leaf
- 2 tablespoons fresh lemon juice
- 1 teaspoon salt
- 12 (10 inch) flour tortillas
- fresh salsa

DIRECTIONS

- Preheat the oven to 350.

- Place the sweet potatoes in a medium saucepan with the salt and water to cover.
- Cover and bring to a boil, then simmer until tender, about 10 minutes.
- Drain and set aside.
- While the sweet potatoes are cooking, warm the oil in a medium skillet or saucepan and add the onions, garlic, and chile.
- Cover and cook on medium-low heat, stirring occasionally, until the onions are tender, about 7 minutes.
- Add the cumin and coriander and cook for 2 to 3 minutes longer, stirring frequently.
- Remove from the heat and set aside.
- In a food processor, combine the black beans, cilantro, lemon juice, salt, and cooked sweet potatoes and puree until smooth (or mash the ingredients in a large bowl by hand).
- Transfer the sweet potato mixture to a large mixing bowl and mix in the cooked onions and spices.

- Lightly oil a large baking dish.
- Spoon about 2/3 to 3/4 cup of the filling in the center of each tortilla, roll it up, and place it, seam side down, in the baking dish.
- Cover tightly with foil and bake for about 30 minutes, until piping hot.
- Serve topped with salsa.

NUTRITION INFO

Serving Size: 1 (2933) g

Servings Per Recipe: 1

AMT. PER SERVING	% DAILY VALUE
Calories: 575.2	
Calories from Fat 92 g	16%
Total Fat 10.3 g	15%
Saturated Fat 2.3 g	11%
Cholesterol 0 mg	0%
Sodium 1156.4 mg	48%
Total Carbohydrate 102 g	33%
Dietary Fiber 15.9 g	63%
Sugars 8.7 g	34%
Protein 19.8 g	39%

Slow-Cooker Black Eyed Peas

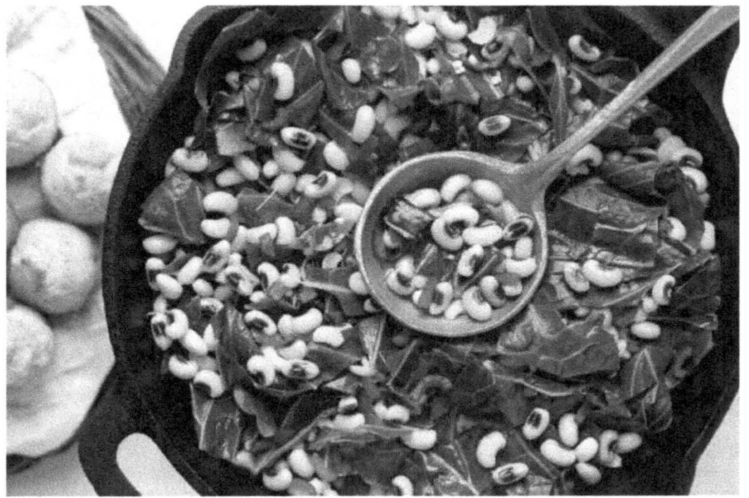

Preparation Time: 9 hours 30 minutes

INGREDIENTS

- 1 (16 ounce) bag dried black-eyed peas
- 1 small ham hock
- 1 (14 1/2 ounce) can Del Monte zesty jalapeno pepper diced tomato
- 1 (14 1/2 ounce) can diced tomatoes with green chilies
- 2 (10 1/2 ounce) cans chicken broth

- 1 stalk celery, chopped

DIRECTIONS

- Pre-soak black-eyed peas according to the instructions on the bag.
- Combine all ingredients and cook on low for 9-10 hours.

NUTRITION INFO

Serving Size: 1 (257) g

Servings Per Recipe: 6

AMT. PER SERVING	% DAILY VALUE
Calories: 282.5	
Calories from Fat 14 g	5%
Total Fat 1.6 g	2%
Saturated Fat 0.4 g	2%
Cholesterol 0 mg	0%
Sodium 618.8 mg	25%
Total Carbohydrate 48.5 g	16%
Dietary Fiber 8.1 g	32%
Sugars 5.7 g	22%
Protein 20.5 g	40%

Sweet Potato Curry With Spinach & Chickpeas

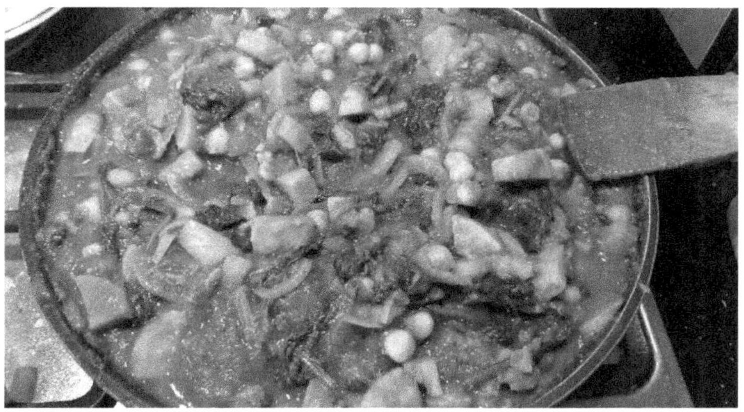

Preparation Time: 27 minutes

INGREDIENTS

- 1⁄2 large sweet onions, chopped or 2 scallions, thinly sliced
- 1 -2 teaspoon canola oil
- 2 tablespoons curry powder
- 1 tablespoon cumin
- 1 teaspoon cinnamon
- 10 ounces fresh spinach, washed, stemmed and coarsely chopped

- 2 large sweet potatoes, peeled and diced (about 2 lbs)
- 1 (14 1/2 ounce) can chickpeas, rinsed and drained
- 1⁄2 cup water
- 1 (14 1/2 ounce) can diced tomatoes, can substitute fresh if available
- 1⁄4 cup chopped fresh cilantro, for garnish
- basmati rice or brown rice, for serving

DIRECTIONS

- You may choose to cook the sweet potatoes however you prefer.
- I like to peel, chop and steam mine in a veggie steamer for about 15 minutes.
- Baking or boiling work well too.
- While sweet potatoes cook, heat 1-2 tsp of canola or vegetable oil over medium heat.
- Add onions and sauté 2-3 minutes, or until they begin to soften.

- Next, add the curry powder, cumin, and cinnamon, and stir to coat the onions evenly with spices.
- Add tomatoes with their juices, and the chickpeas, stir to combine.
- Add ½ cup water and raise heat up to a strong simmer for about a minute or two.
- Next, add the fresh spinach, a couple handfuls at a time, stirring to coat with cooking liquid.
- When all the spinach is added to the pan, cover and simmer until just wilted, about 3 minutes.
- Add the cooked sweet potatoes to the liquid, and stir to coat.
- Simmer for another 3-5 minutes, or until flavors are well combined.
- Transfer to serving dish, toss with fresh cilantro, and serve hot.
- This dish is nice served over basmati or brown rice.

NUTRITION INFO

Serving Size: 1 (269) g

Servings Per Recipe: 6

AMT. PER SERVING	% DAILY VALUE
Calories: 166.5	
Calories from Fat 21 g	13%
Total Fat 2.4 g	3%
Saturated Fat 0.3 g	1%
Cholesterol 0 mg	0%
Sodium 277.5 mg	11%
Total Carbohydrate 32 g	10%
Dietary Fiber 7.5 g	30%
Sugars 4.5 g	17%
Protein 6.8 g	13%

French Vanilla Almond Granola

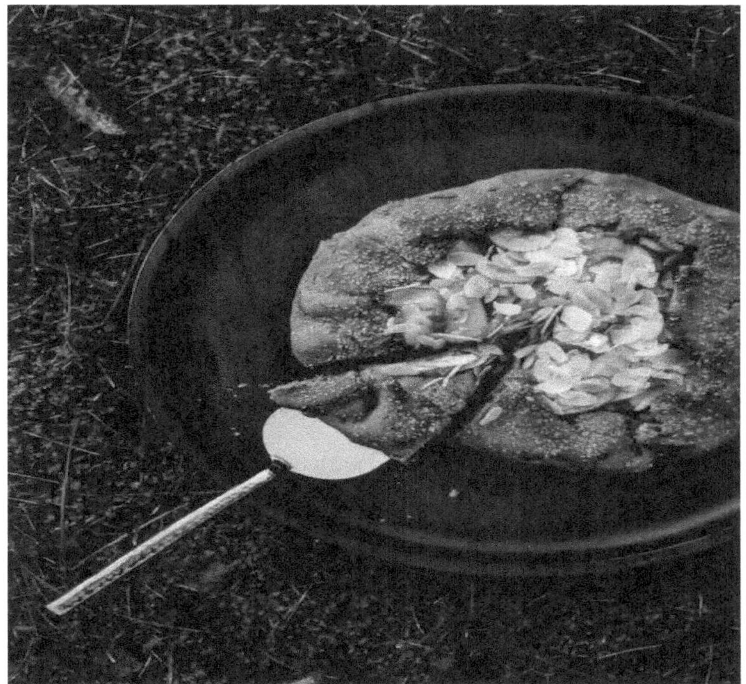

Preparation Time: 120 minutes

INGREDIENTS

- 3 1⁄2 cups old fashioned oats (not quick)
- 1⁄2 cup sliced almonds
- 1⁄2 cup water
- 1⁄2 cup natural cane sugar

- 1⁄4 teaspoon salt
- 1⁄4 cup organic canola oil or 1/4 cup grapeseed oil
- 1 tablespoon vanilla extract

DIRECTIONS

- ➢ Heat oven to 200 degrees F. Line a large, rimmed cookie sheet with parchment paper.
- ➢ In a large bowl mix together the oats and almonds.
- ➢ In a small saucepan over medium heat, stir the sugar and salt into the water. Cook and stir until sugar is dissolved. Remove from heat. Stir in canola oil and vanilla. Pour into the oat and almond mixture and stir until thoroughly combined.
- ➢ Spread mixture out on the lined cookie sheet and bake for 2 hours, or until dry to the touch. Do not stir! Remove from oven and let cool before breaking apart into chunks. Store in an air-tight container.

NUTRITION INFO

Serving Size: 1 (51) g

Servings Per Recipe: 12

AMT. PER SERVING	% DAILY VALUE
Calories: 187.1	
Calories from Fat 71 g	38%
Total Fat 8 g	12%
Saturated Fat 0.7 g	3%
Cholesterol 0 mg	0%
Sodium 50.4 mg	2%
Total Carbohydrate 25.3 g	8%
Dietary Fiber 2.9 g	11%
Sugars 8.8 g	35%
Protein 3.9 g	7%

Poached Eggs & Avocado Toasts

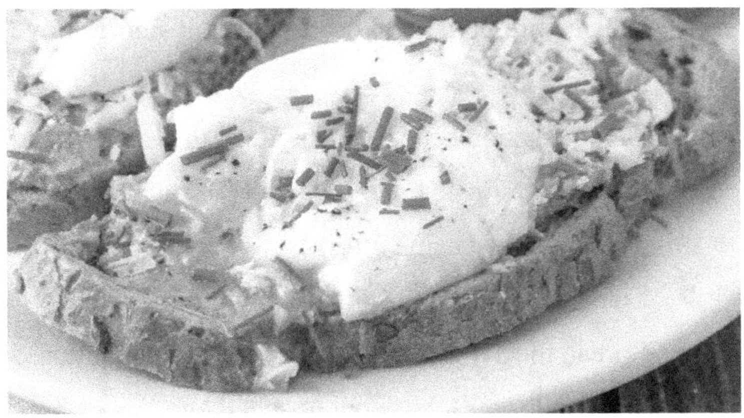

Preparation Time: 12 minutes

INGREDIENTS

- 4 eggs
- 2 ripe avocados
- 2 teaspoons lemon juice (or juice of 1 lime)
- 4 slices thick bread
- 1 cup cheese (grated, edam, gruyere or whatever you have on hand)
- salt & freshly ground black pepper
- 4 teaspoons butter (for spreading on toast)

DIRECTIONS

- Poach eggs using your favourite method.
- Meanwhile cut the avocados in half and remove the stones.
- Using a spoon scoop out the flesh into a bowl and add the lemon or lime juice and the salt & pepper.
- Mash roughly using a fork.
- Toast the bread and spread with butter.
- Spread the avocado mix onto each slice of buttered toast and top each with a poached egg.

- Sprinkle over the grated cheese and serve immediately.
- These are also nice with either fresh or grilled tomato halves on the side.

NUTRITION INFO

Serving Size: 1 (216) g

Servings Per Recipe: 4

AMT. PER SERVING	% DAILY VALUE
Calories: 439.8	
Calories from Fat 280 g	64%
Total Fat 31.2 g	47%
Saturated Fat 10.7 g	53%
Cholesterol 214.2 mg	71%
Sodium 537.7 mg	22%
Total Carbohydrate 26.6 g	8%
Dietary Fiber 7.5 g	29%
Sugars 2.2 g	8%
Protein 16.2 g	31%

Millet & Quinoa Mediterranean Salad

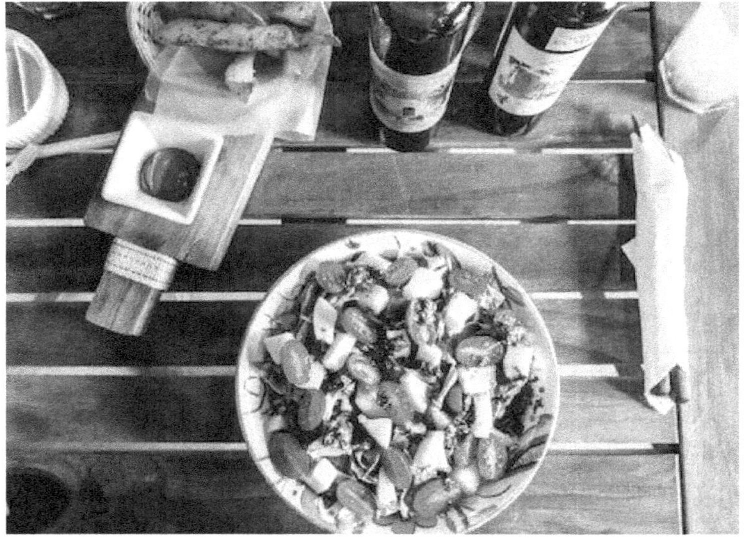

Preparation Time: 35 minutes

INGREDIENTS

- 1⁄2 cup millet
- 1 cup water
- 1⁄2 cup quinoa (red, white, or black)
- 3⁄4 cup water
- 1 English cucumber, diced
- 1 tomatoe, ripe, seeds squeezed out, diced

- 1 sweet pepper, seeded, diced
- 1⁄2 red onion, sliced thin
- 1 garlic clove, pressed
- 200g feta cheese, diced
- 1 (10 ounce) can large white beans, drained
- 1⁄4 teaspoon cayenne pepper (more, to taste)
- 2 teaspoons dried dill (sub basil or oregano, if preferred)
- 1⁄4 cup pine nuts
- 1 lemon, juice of (zest as well, if preferred)
- 1 tablespoon olive oil (optional)
- fresh ground pepper, to taste

DIRECTIONS

- ➢ Bring millet and 1 cup water to boil, reduce heat, and simmer for five minutes; turn off heat, cover, and let sit for 10 minutes.
- ➢ Bring quinoa and 3/4 cup water to boil, reduce heat, and simmer, covered, for 12-14 minutes; fluff.
- ➢ Combine all ingredients and toss; chill. Enjoy

CONCLUSION

After consulting various researches and studies on the positive effects of fasting, the results have proven to be quite convincing. It is, therefore, safe to say that intermittent fasting is indeed a reasonable medical intervention for women over 50 who either want to lose weight or are looking for improved overall health by keeping diseases at bay.

Intermittent fasting generally is a safe and healthy way to lose weight and combat numerous diseases just by keeping a check on the timing during which you consume your daily calories.

For women over 50, intermittent fasting is a way out of their medical issues such as obesity, arthritis, joint pain, mental health issues, diabetes, blood pressure, so on and so forth. These health conditions are quite damaging in the long run; therefore, it is better to prevent them rather than allow them to cause you pain and discomfort along with the monetary burden they bring. Intermittent fasting is a highly advisable technique that women over 50 or even under 50 should incorporate into their lifestyle rather than adopting it as a diet for the short term. After all, prevention is better than cure!

www.ingramcontent.com/pod-product-compliance
Lightning Source LLC
LaVergne TN
LVHW050603160826
845677LV00011B/2441

* 9 7 9 8 3 5 2 5 8 8 6 9 7 *